The Goddess's Guide
To Women's
Health

Purple Rose Ink Publications

ISBN-13: 978-1542692656

ISBN-10: 1542692652

Table of Contents

Introduction

Over the years, I've collected information about health, but women's health in particular. Much of the information I collected was collected in an effort to understand how my anatomy worked and to understand the vague, but troubling symptoms I suffered from.

Some of the information came from Health Class in High School as well the Home Economics Class and the Kids, Kids, Kids. Some of the information came from my college Human Health Class.

The bulk of the information came from books I read and the internet though. Until I had finally had children of my own and got on Medicaid, I was frequently without health insurance. This meant that I couldn't go to the doctor and get the tests I needed. Really, I couldn't rely on Western Medicine to help me get healthy and conceive the baby I wanted. So, I went back to my roots.

I found myself interested in Herbs and Holistic Health around 12 years of age. I once had dreams of owning my own Herb Shop and being able to prescribe herbs to those in need. As I got older, my interest faded but never completely went away. When I had trouble conceiving, I returned to my interest in holistic health. I researched what herbs to take to help with conception and which ones I should avoid so that I didn't have a miscarriage. I discovered what ones are safe to take once I finally conceived as well.

Eventually, I did get pregnant. I am not sure that the herbs helped, but I can say that certainly didn't hurt. I was sure that I had a hormonal imbalance, but had no way to test myself. Taking natural estrogen didn't seem to help me. In fact, it seemed to make things worse. When I started taking Vitex or Chasteberry and using Progesterone cream, I finally found some regularity and relief from my painful cycles. Later, when I went to the doctor for tests to see if I had a hormonal imbalance, they merely tested for testosterone. I was greatly frustrated that they didn't check for estrogen dominance or a lack of progesterone.

Between the birth of my daughter and the birth of my son, I had Medicaid, so I was able get a bunch of tests I couldn't otherwise afford. These tests revealed that I had been born with a genetic defect. I had a small, misshapen uterus and two ovaries, but only one fallopian tube. My right ovary was normal, but my left was attached my pelvic wall and did not reach my uterus at all. It would be reasonable to assume that this irregularity cut my chances of conceiving in half and could potentially have been responsible for my irregular periods.

So why the title this Women's Health Book *The Goddess's Guide*? Well, I wanted this book to be a celebration a women and Wicca does just that. I began reading about Wicca in High School and then some more in college. Many women who were natural healers in the past were deemed to be witches. I wanted to embrace the label of witch and the idea the women were once honored in Goddess worship.

Chapter 1: Anatomy

I found the best book on Woman's Anatomy is the poetic *Woman: An Intimate Geography* by Natalie Angier. The 1999 book breaks down the female anatomy and explores gender stereotypes. I would suggest picking up her book for a more detailed account, but I would like to give you a brief overview of how our bodies work here.

The egg is where it all begins. Women produce eggs in their ovaries. Surprisingly women are born with all the eggs they will ever have and we have potentially millions of them. By the time we begin ovulating in puberty that number will have dropped into the thousands. Where do the eggs go? Why, they are systematically destroyed by the body in a process called Apoptosis. What is left over can drop down through the fallopian tube for fertilization. What causes the egg to drop?

We have several hormones that work with our body to help us reproduce. Important Hormones to be aware of are: Testosterone, Estrogen, Progesterone, Prolactin, Cortisol and DHEA.

Believe it or not, women have Testosterone just the same as men, although in much lower levels. It is testosterone that is responsible for our sex drive. Though we already have some in our bodies, men transfer a bit to us through their saliva when we kiss. This makes us more inclined to sleep with them!

Prolactin is the hormone released in order to trigger lactation. This happens when we get pregnant. Prolactin also suppress ovulation when breastfeeding. This means that breastfeeding can be a sort of natural birth control. However, it is not 100% reliable. Most doctors won't recommend it for women. Instead, they will want you to use condoms or go on the pill—the progesterone only pill, since it safe to use while breastfeeding.

The buildup in Estrogen and Progesterone levels do rigger changes in our cycle, but it is the hypothalamus that first releases the *gonadotropin-releasing hormone (GnRH) and the* luteinizing hormone (LH). Then there is the follicle-stimulating hormone (FSH) that is released and that actually stimulate the ovary into giving up its egg that month.

Estrogen and Progesterone build up, the lining of the uterus thickens and the body prepares for pregnancy. Ovulation takes place around day 14 of the cycle, after your hormone peak. If you are planning to get pregnant, the experts suggest having sex around day 12 since sperm can live inside a woman for up to 72 hours. Anyway, if the egg is not fertilized then the hormonal levels drop and the lining of the uterus is shed. A normal menstrual cycle is anywhere from 21 to 28 days. However, it can vary anywhere from 21 days to 45 days in some women.

As a teen, I was never like clockwork. It varied from month to month, but only by a few days. I went on birth control briefly and went off of it. I had to go back on when I started having extremely heavy painful periods every 14 days or so. Due to lack of insurance, I had to go to Planned Parenthood for my birth control pills. They gave and exam and birth control on a sliding scale fee, which was helpful. However, they didn't really listen to me or help with my complicated issues. In any case, when I went off birth control some years later, I would have a 14 day cycle followed by a 45 day cycle. It was more than a little frustrating, to say the least. And it made it difficult to predict ovulation.

Chapter 2: PMS

PMS stands for Premenstrual Syndrome. About one to two weeks before your period, you may experience tender breasts, bloating, cramps, mood swings, and headaches. About 85% of women experience some of the symptoms during their lifetime. Symptoms may be mild in some women, while others are debilitated by the severity of them.

What causes PMS? Being overweight, stressed out and eating poorly can all contribute to PMS, but generally, it is thought be the result of hormonal changes in the body. As hormone levels drop, our bodies react. There appears to be less serotonin in the brain after ovulation, which is why medications like Prozac can be used to elevate mood when PMS strikes.

PMDD or Premenstrual Dysphoria Disorder is a severe form of PMS. When a woman loses all energy and is severely depressed before her period, a diagnosis of PMDD may be made. Only about 3% to 8% of women actually have it though. Usually there is an underlying condition of Major Depression, made worse by fluctuating hormones.

Multivitamins, turmeric, evening primrose oil and fish oil are recommended to minimize the effects of PMS. Many women find that their symptoms lessen when they regulate their hormones with birth control, but not all.

Chapter 3: History of Birth Control

Over 75 percent women take birth control at some point in their lives, but most don't realize the long hard fight that it took to get birth control available to us with such ease. There have been barrier methods such as condoms and herbal concoctions in use for a long time. But not everyone knew about these methods. It was often the courtesan or prostitute who employed such methods. Most women felt prohibited from preventing pregnancy by their religious beliefs.

Some early Herbal Contraception included: Wild Yam, Neem, Queen Anne's lace, Pomegranate, Rutin, Smartweed Leaves, Apricot Kernels, Rue, Cotton Wood, Bark and more recently, High Dosages of Vitamin C.

Margaret Sanger (September 14, 1879 – September 6, 1966) is considered the founder of Planned Parenthood. Sanger felt that in order for women to have a more equal footing in society and to lead healthier lives, they needed to be able to determine when to bear children. She was prosecuted for her book *Family Limitation* and for distributing information on birth control back in 1916. The 1873 Comstock Law against profanity made any information on sex, reproduction and birth control nearly impossible to access for the common woman. This led to Sanger founding The American Birth Control League and Planned Parenthood in 1921 in order to help women become more educated and be given more options. She strongly believed in the freedom of speech.

Sadly, Sanger is often demonized by antiabortionists. Sanger herself did not agree with the practice, but felt women should have a safe place to go instead of dying from back alley abortions. Her proponents also site the eugenics program as evidence of her racism. However, Sanger never believed in the extreme views on eugenics. She merely felt that people needed to limit the number of children they had.

Although the FDA approved the Pill in 1960, it wasn't until in 1965, the Supreme Court ruled in *Griswold v. Connecticut* that it was unconstitutional for the government to prohibit married couples from using birth control. Soon, single women were also able to obtain birth control as well.

When I took Home Economics in High School back in 1991, we were given a sheet with birth control methods available to us. Options have changed quite a bit since then. Women can use the estrogen and progesterone pill, the progesterone only pill, Depo-Provera shot, the Norplant implant, the Nuvaring and the Patch. The IUD was available for a while, was taken off the market and then reintroduced in a safer version. Sponges, Spermicides and Condoms are also options. One popular spermicide is the Vaginal Film Contraceptive or VCF. Though not particularly popular, there is also the female condom available as well.

Some women, me included, can be allergic or sensitive to spermicide. If you get a bad yeast infection after using a condom with spermicide this can be why. You may have to make sure to get condoms without spermicide on them. They maybe be a tad less effective, but it will save you a lot misery in the long run.

Did you know that the first condoms were called The English Overcoat and were made way back in the 1500s? They were often made of lambskin. Vulcanized rubber in the 1840s made condoms more accessible and convenient for men. It was until 1985 that the first commercial for condoms appeared on TV. During the 1980s, when AIDS was a huge concern, condoms became the first line of defense. They are no longer one size fits all and come in many shapes and sizes.

Chapter 4: Sexually Transmitted Infections

Common diseases include: HIV/AIDS, Bacterial Vaginosis, Chlamydia, Gonorrhea, Genital Warts, HPV, Syphilis, Trichomoniasis, Pelvic Inflammatory Disease, Pubic Lice, Hepatitis and UTI. Keep in mind that you can not only get Sexually Transmitted Diseases from unprotected intercourse, but from anal or oral sex as well.

HPV can cause vaginal cancer. There is now an immunization for both men and women that helps eliminate this virus. Though not all people with HPV develop cancer, there is definitely a connection between the two. It certainly increases your chance of cancer if you have HPV.

Untreated diseases can lead to Pelvic Inflammatory Disease, which can cause infertility. I had a friend who got Chlamydia from her cheating husband and didn't get it treated right away. Then she was re-infected when her husband didn't take his medicine. This caused PID and now she is unable to have children due to the scarring and adhesions she has. So, if you want to have children, it is important to make sure you stay on top of any unusual itches, pain or rashes. Also make sure to get routine check-ups because some infections, like Chlamydia, don't always present symptoms.

Chlamydia, Gonorrhea and Syphilis are all fairly common infections. Usually they are easily treated with antibiotics—even Syphilis, which used to be fatal. However, sometimes the both the disease and the antibiotics to treat it can cause a miscarriage in pregnant women. But it is better to treat the disease than risk, not only miscarriage, but serious complications for the pregnant woman

Pregnant women are often screen for specific troublesome diseases. They may test for Strep B, Rubella, Gestational Diabetes, Urinary Tract Infections, Diabetes, High Blood Pressure and Preeclampsia. Often not on the doctor's radar, but potentially dangerous, are: Gallbladder Disease, Liver Disease, Rheumatoid Arthritis, Autoimmune Disease, Fibromyalgia, Asthma, Meningitis, Cancer and Preterm Labor.

Chapter 5: UTI

Urinary Tract infections are common in women. They happen more frequently in sexually active women, but there plenty of women who get them without being sexually active. Signs of a urinary tract infection are: flank pain, high fever, chills, vomiting, a burning sensation while urinating and increased frequency of urination.

Cystitis is commonly known as a bladder infection. It can be caused by frequent or rough intercourse, but it can also come from wiping improperly after a bowel movement, particularly diarrhea. The infection comes from bacteria, usually E Coli, which enters the urethra and causes inflammation and infection.

Urethritis is an infection of urethra, not just the bladder. Sometimes it can be hard to diagnosis since there isn't always large amounts of bacteria present in the urine. E Coli and Chlamydia are two of the most common culprits.

A kidney infection can become quite serious if left untreated. A kidney infection happens when the bacteria travels from the bladder, up the urethra and into the kidneys. Antibiotics are used to treat all UTIs. Macrobid (Nitrofurantoin) is the most common antibiotic used.

Personally, I had trouble with UTIs for a while. It seemed like once I got the infection, I couldn't get rid of it entirely. I took my antibiotics and felt better, only to get another infection a short time later. I read that once E Coli gets into the bladder and urethra, it is difficult to get it all out. The first time I got pregnant, I went to the doctor to treat the UTI and found out I was pregnant as well. Unfortunately, I miscarried a short time later. UTIs are common in pregnancy though.

You can treat UTIs with over the counter AZO Urinary Pain Relief, which contains phenazopyridine hydrochloride. That will help with the burning. It is recommended that you avoid caffeine and drink as much water as possible during an infection. Cranberry Juice has been proven to help get rid of the infection. It prevents the bacteria from attaching to the wall of your bladder. If you can't stand the tart taste of cranberry juice, then there are now cranberry pills available.

Chapter 6: Mental Health

Everyone feels down or depressed at times. Having a major depressive episode is more than just being sad for a while. You may also feel anxiety, apathy, general discontent, guilt, hopelessness, loss of interest, loss of interest or pleasure in activities and have mood swings. Usually sleep patterns are disturbed with early awakening, excess sleepiness, insomnia, or restless sleep being common issues. Depression may result in either lack of appetite and weight loss or increased hunger and weight gain. While many women find themselves in tears constantly, others get irritable and downright angry at times. Thoughts of self-harm and suicide can occur as well.

While depression is the most prevalent disorder, some women find themselves with other symptoms that lead to different or additional diagnoses. Being Bipolar or Manic Depressive can resembled being depressed in many ways. However, in addition to feeling depressed there are manic episodes. Manic episodes may be marked by periods of great excitement, euphoria, delusions, and over activity. In its extreme thoughts may race and obsessions may develop. When it is mild, mania may take the form of anxiety. The most dangerous state is what they call a mixed state—when one is both depressed and anxious at the same time.

Borderline Personality Disorder is not as common, but it often overlaps with signs of Depression and/or Bipolar disorder.

Depression, anxiety and feelings of worthlessness are symptoms, but what sets it BPD apart from the others is extreme anger, unstable relationships and impulsive actions. Heightened paranoia about being abandoned and self-harm occur more with BPD than other disorders. Women who have been the victim of abuse are more likely to develop this disorder. Unfortunately, the women with BPD are also more likely to continue the cycle of abuse and hurt others because of their pasts and their disorder.

Treatment for these three disorders and others require evaluation by a doctor or psychiatrist. Medication and talk therapy are common ways to address the symptoms. There are herbs that be used to elevate some of the feelings, but they should be used cautiously. Herbal supplements can interact with certain medications and have unwanted side effects. Be sure to discuss any herbal supplements you are taking with your doctor.

Valerian is a safe and natural alternative to sleep medication. Melatonin can also be used to regulate sleepy cycles. St John's Wart has often been used to help elevated depression, however, it can interfere with the pill and make it less effective.

SAMe or S-adenosyl-L-methionine is a compound made naturally by the body and is now available as dietary supplement. SAMe helps produce serotonin, melatonin, and dopamine and may help with osteoarthritis, heart disease, ADHD and epilepsy in addition to depression.

Vitamins B, C and E can all help the body function better and improve symptoms of depression. Omega Fish Oils are also recommended for depression as well as heart health. GABA or *Gamma*-Aminobutyric Acid is a natural amino acid found in our bodies, but it can also be taken as a supplement for anxiety.

Chapter 7: Domestic Violence

Domestic Violence can happen to anyone. It doesn't matter what race, class or sex you are. It happens to both men and women who are rich, poor, black, white, gay or straight. It is often physical, but it doesn't have to be. Domestic violence is almost never just about hurting someone physically. In almost all abusive relationships, physical abuse is accompanied by emotional manipulation and verbal abuse. The verbal and emotional abuse are tool that allow the abuser to keep power and control over his or her victim.

How do you know if you are being abused? It isn't always obvious or easy to spot, but if you ask yourself these questions, it might help make things clearer for you.

Does your partner embarrass or make fun of you in front of friends or family? Does your partner put down your accomplishments or goals? Does your partner make you feel like you are unable to make decisions? Do they used intimidation or threats to gain your compliance? Does your partner tell you that you are nothing without them? Do they treat you roughly by grabbing, pushing, pinching, shoving or hitting you? Does your partner call you several times a day or show up to make to sure you are where you said you'd be? Do they blame you for how they feel or act? Does your partner use drugs or alcohol as an excuse for saying hurtful things or for hurting you? Do they make you feel like there is no way out of the relationship? Does your partner prevent you from doing things you want like spending time with your friends and family? Do they try to keep you from leaving after a fight?

Do you sometimes feel scared of how your partner will act? Do you constantly make excuses to other people for your partner's behavior? Do you believe that you can help your partner change only if you changed something about yourself? Do you try to not do anything to make your partner angry? Do you feel like no matter what you do your partner is never happy with you? Do you always do what your partner wants you to do instead of what you want? Do you stay with your partner because you are afraid of what your partner would do if you broke up?

If you answered yes to some or all these questions then you may need to seek some help to deal with your situation. Some women think because they hit back that it is okay, but violence is never okay. The best thing to do is get out of the abusive relationship and remove yourself from harm's way. If you don't have friends or family members to turn to for help, there are women's shelters that can help. Counseling may also be an important step in not only helping you take action, but in healing from the damage done. If you are unsure where to turn to or what to do next, you can always call the Domestic Violence Hotline at 1-800-799-7233.

When you get involved in a new relationship, make sure start things off on the right foot. Set boundaries, establish trust and try to communicate clearly from the get go. Make sure they never do anything without your consent. Don't let anyone take advantage of you or force you to do anything you don't want to do.

Chapter 8: Thyroid

Thyroid Issues can wreak havoc on a women's life as well. The thyroid is small gland along the throat. However, it is very important for maintaining a balance in the body. If the Thyroid is underactive or overactive either one, it can make you miserable.

Hyperthyroidism, also known as Grave's Disease, is when the thyroid is overactive. Symptoms include losing weight, weakness, irregular heartbeat, and difficulty sleeping.

Hypothyroidism is an underactive thyroid. Symptoms include: exhaustion, hair loss or dryness, brittle nails, constipation, dry skin, enlarged thyroid, high cholesterol, irritability, sensitivity to cold, sexual dysfunction, slow heart rate, sluggishness, weight gain, or irregular uterine bleeding.

What causes an underactive thyroid? Pesticides, heavy metal poisoning and chronic stress can all trigger an imbalance. Chronic inflammation caused by grain or gluten can also contribute. Pain medications, antihistamines and antidepressants can also slow down your thyroid too.

There are those that they theorize that Hypothyroidism is rooted in an immune system gone crazy. Unfortunately, most doctors won't treat the problem unless it is severe, but there are ways you can improve your thyroid function naturally.

Avoid caffeine, sugar, carbs, fluoride and nonstick cookware. Eat protein and get your Omega-3 fats. Natural, healthy fats include olive oil, nuts, fish, cheese and yogurts. Also taking supplements can help as well. Vitamin D, Iron, Omega-3, Zinc, Copper, Vitamin A, Vitamin B and Iodine can all help.

Chapter 9: Hypertension

Hypertension or High Blood Pressure Blood is determined by the amount of blood your heart pumps and the amount of resistance to blood flow in your arteries. The more blood your heart pumps and the narrower your arteries, the higher your blood pressure.

There is often no signs of high blood pressure. It may gradually build up over years and years before it is recognized or caught. Because there are rarely signs, you might not know you have it until you go to the doctor and have it checked.

Sometimes there is no underlying cause, but there are other medical conditions that can cause high blood pressure. Obstructive sleep apnea, kidney problems, adrenal gland tumors, thyroid problems and certain defects in blood vessels you're born with can all increase blood pressure. Things like birth control pills, cold remedies, decongestants, over-the-counter pain relievers and some prescription drugs, illegal drugs well as alcohol abuse or chronic alcohol use can increase blood pressure as well.

The older you are, the more at risk you are for developing high blood pressure. Genetics and environmental factors also play role. Diet is very important because too much salt and not enough potassium in your diet is enough to gradually elevate your blood pressure over time. A Vitamin D deficiency can also elevate your blood pressure, which can be a problem for night shift workers. Stress, especially chronic stress, will contribute to heart disease too.

If hypertension is left untreated, it can cause a wide range of problems, including: memory loss, vision loss, metabolic syndrome stroke, aneurysm heart attack, heart failure and kidney failure.

Metabolic Syndrome is syndrome is a cluster of disorders of your body's metabolism, including increased waist circumference, high triglycerides, low good cholesterol; high blood pressure and high insulin levels.

Usually doctors will recommend trying improve your diet—especially cutting back on salt. If diet and exercise don't improve your blood pressure numbers, then they will put you on medication to keep under control. They may prescribe diuretics, ACE inhibitors, ARBs, calcium channel blockers, beta blockers or vasodilators to help.

Natural approaches to lowing blood pressure include increasing fiber in your diet. Taking minerals supplements such as magnesium, calcium, potassium and folic acid can help. Things such as cocoa, coenzyme Q10, L-arginine or garlic, Omega-3 fatty acids and flaxseed are natural vasodilators and they can help as well.

Meditation and Yoga have been shown to lower stress and thus lower blood pressure. Anything you can do to relax and take care of yourself is helpful.

Chapter 10: Strokes

Strokes occur due to problems with the blood supply to the brain: either the blood supply is blocked or a blood vessel within the brain ruptures, causing brain tissue to die due to lack of oxygen. A stroke is a medical emergency, and treatment must be sought as quickly as possible.

What are the signs you are having a stroke? Early signs are Bladder or bowel control problems, depression, pain in the hands and feet that gets worse with movement and temperature changes, paralysis or weakness on one or both sides of the body and trouble controlling or expressing emotions. More severe symptoms include: confusion, trouble with speaking and understanding, headache, possibly with altered consciousness or vomiting, numbness of the face, arm or leg, particularly on one side of the body, trouble with seeing, in one or both eyes and trouble with walking, including dizziness and lack of co-ordination.

The acronym **F.A.S.T.** is a way to remember the signs of stroke, and can help identify the onset of stroke more quickly: **F**ace drooping: if the person tries to smile does one side of the face droop? **A**rm weakness: if the person tries to raise both their arms does one arm drift downward? **S**peech difficulty: if the person tries to repeat a simple phrase is their speech slurred or strange? **T**ime to call 911: if any of these signs are observed, contact the emergency services.

There are many risk factors involved with strokes. Smoking cigarettes, being overweight or being obese, sleep apnea, high blood pressure, high cholesterol, diabetes and heart disease can all contribute to the occurrence of a stroke. The highest stroke rates are among African American males over 55, but women have them too. Even if you don't fit into any of the other categories, you can still have a stroke if you are doing Meth or Coke or even just drinking heavily for a long time.

There is no cure for a stroke, but there are herbal supplements you can take to decrease your risks. Bilberry may improve cholesterol and lower blood sugar. Garlic may prevent blood clotting and destroy plaque. Ginkgo may improve blood flow to the brain and Asian ginseng may improve memory and decreases diabetes risk. Black Tea and Green Tea are also supposed to be helpful. Eating more fruit is good—particularly pomegranate. Vitamins B, C, D and E in addition to Magnesium are recommended as well.

Getting to the hospital as quickly as possible is the key to preventing irreversible damage or death. However, even in the best of circumstances road to recovery is often a long and difficult one. Physical therapy and speech therapy may be needed. And not all motor functions may return. Memory loss and cognitive issues may arise. If you suffer a stroke, you may need help doing daily things like getting dressed—either right after the stroke or even for the rest of your life. A stroke is life changing and can be debilitating, which is why it is vital to be on top of things and take preventative measures.

Chapter 11: Migraines

Migraines aren't just headaches—they can be intense and debilitating. Though both men and women get migraines, women are much more likely to suffer from them. Tension is leading cause of normal headaches and while stress can trigger a migraine, the nature of the pain much more complicated. Migraines are caused by the swelling of the blood vessels and the nerves. The brain becomes hypersensitive and serotonin levels drop.

How can you tell the difference between a normal headache and a migraine? A migraine will be accompanied by moderate to severe pain on one side of the head. It may feel like stabbing pain in the back of one eye. The pain will get worse while doing activities or even just bending down. There may or may not be a visual aura. The pain will throb and pulsate. There may also be increased sensitivity to light and sound as well as nausea.

It is hereditary to some degree, but migraines are often triggered by women's hormonal changes. Using birth control can increase migraines. Some medicines, like antibiotics, can cause migraines. Weather changes and high altitudes can contribute. However, stress is probably one of the biggest triggers.

There are many treatments today, including the prescription drug Zomig. Herbs can help as well. Though there is no cure, but

Feverfew, Fish Oil, Chamomile, Butter Bur, B2 and Magnesium can help cut down on the intensity and frequency of migraines.

Chapter 12: Sinuses

Sometimes chronic sinusitis can trigger migraines, but mostly they are a pain all on their own. Colds and Sinus infections can make the lining of the sinuses become red and inflamed and cause acute sinusitis.   Allergies can cause chronic inflammation.

Symptoms of Sinusitis are pain around the eyes or cheeks, congestion on one or both sides of the nose, headaches that can be severe, fever, difficulty breathing through the nose and sometimes even toothaches. The treatment for sinusitis is usually over the counter decongestants and prescription antibiotics. You have watch though, because decongestants can increase blood pressure.

When I was on birth control and suffering from a lot of allergy, sinus and migraine issues, I found out the hard way that decongestants can make things worse. When I had a migraine decongestants only increased the pain because it increased my blood pressure. If you think your sinus pain has turned into a migraine consider taking Benadryl or some sort of allergy medicine and take a hot shower instead of relying on decongestants. I do take decongestant, but only when I have a cold or the flu. I never take it for everyday allergy and sinus problems.

Sometimes when antibiotics don't work, surgery may be necessary.

Chapter: 13: Hypoglycemia

What is Hypoglycemia? It is low blood sugar. The normal range for sugar in the blood is 60 mg/dl to 120 mg/dl. Blood sugar levels below 45 mg/dl are always cause for concern. Glucose, which is a form of sugar, is the body's main fuel.

Hypoglycemia occurs when the levels of glucose drop too low to properly fuel the body's needs. Carbohydrates are the body's main sources glucose. The pancreas is in charge of producing insulin and glucagon, but sometimes the body absorbs too much of the sugar and levels in the blood drop below optimal levels for functioning perfectly.

Symptoms of Hypoglycemia are weakness, drowsiness, confusion, hunger, paleness, headache, irritability, trembling, sweating, rapid heartbeat and feeling cold.

Usually Hypoglycemia is a byproduct of Diabetes. However, there are those who suffers from Hypoglycemia who do not have Diabetes. Hypoglycemia not related to Diabetes is usually connected to have not enough cortisol in your system. People with Addison's disease, for example, will not have enough glucagon, or not enough epinephrine, which can result in low blood sugar.

I've have never been diagnosed with it diabetes nor have I been diagnosed with Hypoglycemia, but I know that I still have issue with blood sugar. I get extremely tired and grumpy if I don't eat. Hangry is a good way to describe it. It is better if I snack or have several small meals in order to function at my best.

Where there is no other obvious causes, low blood sugar maybe connected to a sugary diet. This is often termed reactive hypoglycemia. If you eat or drink something sugary and crash afterward, you may want to avoid that particular food or drink. I believe you can be sensitive to sugar or particular types of sugars in food even if it is not severe enough to be diagnosed as Hypoglycemia.

Another possible cause of Hypoglycemia is birth control pills. I know when I was on a high dose of estrogen that my blood sugar issues became more severe. This was because the higher levels of estrogen in your body, the more Cortisol is released. Your adrenal glands can become exhausted and you can suffer from hormone induced Hypoglycemia.

Chapter 14: Diabetes

Diabetes happens when the body, particularly the pancreas, doesn't produce enough insulin and there is too much sugar in the blood. There are two types of Diabetes that can occur.

Type 1 Diabetes is usually something you are born with or develop at a young age. It is actually pretty rare. Doctors don't know what causes it, but they do know that genetics plays a role. The only way to treat Type 1 Diabetes is daily insulin injections.

Type 2 Diabetes is far more common. It develops largely because of lifestyle and diet issues. Depression, weight, age and cholesterol levels all factor in. Smoking is a big risk factor as well. However, the biggest factor is probably diet. If you eat a lot of processed sugars, carbohydrates and fats then this can wreak havoc on the body. Eventually your body fails to keep up with the high demand on it to process these foods and ends up not being able to produce enough insulin.

Symptoms of Diabetes include, heavy thirst, increased hunger especially after eating, dry mouth, nausea and vomiting, pain in your belly, frequent urination, unexplained weight loss, fatigue, blurred vision, heavy or labored breathing, frequent infections of the skin, urinary tract, or vagina.

If untreated it can cause problems with your heart and blood vessels. It can damage your eyes, your kidneys and your nerves. You may notice that wounds stop healing as fast or at all. If you think you might have diabetes get tested and get treatment as soon as possible. Your doctor can get you insulin and/or help you with dietary and lifestyle changes. There is no cure, but it can be managed well.

Chapter 15: Yeast Connection

The Yeast Connection is a book written by William G Crook in 1986. The idea of his book is that Yeast is connected to a lot of our health problems. Chronic Fatigue, depression and other issues can be caused by or made worse by an overgrowth of yeast in the body. A diet rich in sugars and carbohydrates can promote the growth of yeast since yeast feeds on sugar. Hormonal changes and birth control pills can exacerbate an existing problem. Pregnancy, STDs and Diabetes can also factor in.

Constant Yeast Infections are often a sign of an underlying immune system dysfunction. And if your Basel Temperature is 97.4 or 97.6 in the morning it may signal an underactive thyroid.

If you have been antibiotics frequently, used birth control for six months to two years straight and have allergies to smoke and mold, you may have a yeast problem. If you have athletes foot, ring worm or nail fungus you could have a yeast problem.

Symptoms of Yeast overgrowth are: fatigue, depression, headache, numbness or tingling, muscle aches, pain or swelling in your joints, abdominal pain, constipation or diarrhea, bloating, intestinal gas, vaginal itching without an actual yeast infection, cramps, PMS, shaking when hungry, infertility, loss of sexual feeling, bladder infections and hypothyroidism.

The solution? Eat more protein and less carbs and sugars. Eliminating soda from your diet and getting off birth control can also help. Avoiding antibiotics whenever possible and treating your allergies may also improve your yeast situation.

Chapter 16: Grain Brain

David Pearlmutter wrote a book called *The Grain Brain* that came out in 2013. It takes the Yeast Connection a whole new direction, claiming that grain or gluten is the underlying cause of inflammation in the body.

He says the chronic headaches, insomnia, depression, epilepsy, ADHD, schizophrenia, irritable bowel syndrome and arthritis are all influenced by the Grain Brain connection. In fact, he says that Alzheimer's is now being considered a 3rd type of Diabetes. Many of the problems connected to Yeast overgrowth can also be connected to grain and carbs in addition to sugar itself.

One thing to keep in mind is that a gluten allergy is different from Celiac Disease. A person with a gluten allergy may be able to tolerate small amounts of gluten, while people with Celiac Disease can't have any gluten at all. Many people that are sensitive to gluten feel better by cutting back on the breads and pastas, but not everyone needs to avoid them entirely.

Symptoms of a Gluten Allergy are often similar to those in Celiac Disease and may include abdominal pain, diarrhea, constipation, fatigue, bloating, heartburn, bloating, anxiety and anemia. Additional symptoms of a gluten allergy may include: trouble breathing, ulcers in the mouth, asthma, depression, osteoporosis, weight loss, rash, swelling of the lips, irritability and anaphylaxis in severe cases.

Pearlmutter's advice is to eliminate simple carbs, processed and/or packaged foods and the switch to high-quality vegetables and high-quality meat & eggs. It would be ideal to eliminate wheat all together, but this is incredibly difficult to do in the US, as a lot of foods that you wouldn't think had wheat in them do. Barley, oats and rye also contain gluten and should be avoided. Corn and rice are good alternatives.

While I think too much grain can contribute to weight gain and a host of other problems, it seems impractical to avoid them entirely. Unless you have an allergy or Celiac Disease, cutting back will probably suffice.

Chapter 17: Fibromyalgia

What is Fibromyalgia? It is wide spread muscle pain throughout the body and exhaustion. It is still misdiagnosed and misunderstood by many. Like many other things, it is often diagnosed when other things have been ruled out or when is not responsive to traditional treatments. t is thought that Fibromyalgia is caused by amplified pain sensations that affect the way the brain processes pain signals.

Fibromyalgia is not a form of arthritis, which specifically the inflammation of joints and muscles. Fibromyalgia doesn't cause damage to joints or muscles in the same way arthritis does. However, there is a link between fibromyalgia and small-fiber polyneuropathy (SFPN). Meaning, that fibromyalgia can cause nerve damage. There confusion stems from the fact that there does seem to be some overlap between arthritis and fibromyalgia can because both can cause chronic pain and fatigue.

The symptoms of Fibromyalgia include: widespread pain—a constant dull ache that has lasted for at least three months, fatigue, cognitive difficulties which impairs the ability to pay attention and concentrate, depression, headaches, pain or cramping in the lower abdomen,

Those suffering from Fibromyalgia often wake up tired even though they might have had a full night's sleep. The problem is sleep is often interrupted by pain—not to mention that many patients with fibromyalgia have other sleep disorders, such as sleep apnea.

No one knows what causes it for sure, but there seems to be a genetic component. Some researchers theorize that stress or poor physical conditioning are factors in the cause of fibromyalgia. Another theory suggests that very slight damage muscle leads to a never ending cycle of pain and fatigue. Some theorize that inflammation causes nerve damage. Others say that non-celiac gluten sensitivity may be an underlying cause of fibromyalgia symptoms, but further research is needed to prove the connection.

In any case, poor lifestyles choices such being a smoker and being obese may increase the risk of an individual developing fibromyalgia.

Women are much more likely to develop fibromyalgia than are men. Many people who have fibromyalgia also have tension headaches, irritable bowel syndrome, anxiety and depression.

There is really no test to gain a diagnosis for fibromyalgia. Usually, it is a diagnosis given when nothing else can be found to be the cause of the pain. There is no cure, but there are a number of treatments available. Doctors have prescribed Opioids or Pain Medications as well as Lyrica, which specifically targets nerve pain. They also prescribe Antidepressants or SSRI's sometimes. Anti-seizure medications such as Gabapentin has also had some success.

Some alternative treatments for Fibromyalgia include massage therapy, acupuncture and even yoga. Herbal supplements recommended are 5-HTP, which is a building block for the brain chemical serotonin. Low levels of serotonin are associated with depression, so it's believed that raising serotonin levels can lead to a better mood. SAMe is also recommended to improve mood and sleep. It is an amino acid derivative that may boost levels of serotonin and dopamine, another brain chemical. Low levels Magnesium may be linked to fibromyalgia, so you may want to take a supplement. Melatonin is often used in supplements to improve sleep and it may also ease fibromyalgia pain. St. John's Wort is sometimes used to treat certain fibromyalgia symptoms, such as depression.

Chapter 18: Multiple Sclerosis

Multiple Sclerosis is when the immune system attacks the protective sheath or myelin that covers nerve fibers. This causes communication problems between the brain and the rest of the body. Eventually, the disease can cause the nerves themselves to deteriorate or become permanently damaged.

No one knows for sure what causes. It is suspected that it is a combination of genetics and environmental factors may be to blame. Infections and an excess intake of salt may also trigger it. Women, for some reason, are more likely to be diagnosed with Multiple Sclerosis.

Symptoms include; bladder problems, constipation, problems with memory, abstraction, attention, word finding, depression, emotional changes, headaches and hearing loss, fatigue, dizziness, vertigo, problems with balance, head movements may cause electric-shock-like sensations, numbness or weakness, pain or tingling in some parts of the body, itching, sexual dysfunction, muscle spasms , spasticity, tremor, vision problems, gait changes, respiratory or breathing problems, seizures, speech disorders and swallowing problems. Later symptoms that may occur are alterations in perception and thinking, extreme fatigue, heat sensitivity.

There isn't a blood test to diagnosis Multiple Sclerosis, but the doctor may order scans and other tests to rule out infection and other diseases. A lumbar puncture may be necessary as well. Once other things have ruled out, Multiple Sclerosis may be diagnosed.

There is no cure, but there are treatments for the symptoms. Gabapentin may be prescribed to help with nerve pain and corticosteroids may be prescribed to suppress the immune system. Vocational Rehabilitation may be utilized to help the patients figure out what jobs they can perform with their disability and train for them. Once Multiple Sclerosis begins to affect movement, physical therapy may be recommended. Cognitive Therapy may also be necessary.

Chapter 19: Lyme Disease

Lyme disease is caused by the bacteria Borrelia Burgdorferi and is transmitted to humans through the bite of infected blacklegged ticks.

Many of the signs and symptoms of Lyme disease—like inflammation—are a consequence of the immune response to the bacteria. The wide-spread inflammation caused by the infection can cause lasting damage if not caught early on.

Common symptoms include fever, mild to severe headaches, fatigue, and a characteristic skin rash called erythema. Lyme Disease Arthritis usually affects the knees. In a minority of patients, arthritis can occur in other joints, including the ankles, elbows, wrists, hips, and shoulders.

Most people with Lyme disease recover completely with a 2-6 week course of antibiotic treatment. For those who develop other syndromes after their infection is treated, pain medications may provide symptomatic relief.

If it isn't treated right away, there are neurological issues and complications. These complications most often occur in the second stage of Lyme disease and may include: numbness, pain, weakness, paralysis of the facial muscles, visual disturbances, and meningitis symptoms such as fever, stiff neck, and severe headache may occur.

Sometimes Lyme Disease is misdiagnosed as Multiple Scleroses, Depression, Chronic Fatigue Syndrome or Fibromyalgia.

The only way to protect against Lyme disease is to wear protective clothing when spending time outside. Wear long pants when hiking and tuck your pants into your socks. Also make sure to wear a hat and long sleeved shirt. Light colored clothing will help you see the ticks before they attach themselves. Check yourself and your pets after spending time outside as well.

Chapter 19: IBS and IBD

Irritable Bowel Syndrome and Inflammatory Bowel Disease are becoming more prevalent in women than ever before. IBS symptoms include diarrhea, constipation, and abdominal cramps. It seems when doctors don't understand what is causing the disruption and irritation to the digestive track they tend to give it the diagnosis of Irritable Bowel Syndrome. Diet and lifestyle changes can help, but usually don't get rid of the issue entirely.

Inflammatory Bowel Disease is where the digestive track suffers from chronic inflammation. It is an autoimmune disease where the body attacks the healthy lining of the intestines, causing either Crohn's or Ulcerative Colitis. Crohn's occurs anywhere in the digestive track, but is usually located in the upper large intestine. Diarrhea is the most common symptom. Ulcerative Colitis occurs when there is bleeding inside the large intestine in form of ulcers. The ulcers are usually located in the lower part of large intestine and are caused by the body attacking itself.

Though pain may be limited to the digestive track, it may also spread throughout the body as well. During flare ups there may also be swelling in knees, ankles, wrists, elbows and shoulders. Unfortunately, arthritis and rashes are not uncommon in moderate to severe flare ups.

Lately, the idea of leaky gut syndrome has been getting a lot of attention. Leaky Gut Syndrome occurs when the lining of the intestines becomes too permeable and it allows substances to leak into the blood stream that shouldn't be there. Doctors are unsure if this causes IBS and IBD or if Leaky Gut is a symptom of them.

There is no cure, but once there is a diagnosis is made through blood tests and a colonoscopy, then there are treatments available. Aminosalicylates are the first line of defense. They help with mild inflammation, but if you are sensitive to aspirin, they can actually make the symptoms worse. Usually corticosteroids and immune-suppressants will be tried next, but taking them long term can have some serious side effects. Surgery may be necessary, but only in severe cases.

A change in diet can help. Eliminating or cutting down on prepackaged and processed foods may improve symptoms. Taking Fish Oil and Probiotics can also be beneficial. Exercise, Yoga and Acupuncture are also alternative therapies that have had some success as well.

Chapter 21: Gallbladder Disease

Although Gallbladder disease can happen to men and women alike, women are much more likely to have it. The gallbladder is a small organ located under your liver. Your gallbladder's purposes is to store the bile produced by your liver and pass it along to the small intestine. Bile helps you digest fats in your small intestine. Gallstones and other irritants may cause inflammation and even infection.

Symptoms of Gallbladder Disease are extreme pain in the middle of your upper abdomen, fever, chills, nausea and vomiting. I constantly felt like I had indigestion that didn't go away with antacids. Then I began to have attacks with severe nausea and vomiting after meals that were high in fat. Then, finally, the attacks progressed intense pain in my chest hurt. It so bad that I couldn't breathe. I felt like I was having a heart attack, which is when I finally went to the ER and discovered it wasn't my heart, but my gallbladder. I might have gone to the doctor sooner if I'd had health insurance, but I didn't.

Blood tests and an ultrasound are the most common ways to diagnosis a gallbladder problem. Once it has been diagnosed, the doctor will usually prescribe antibiotics. If you have had repeated courses of antibiotics and symptoms haven't improved, then surgery may be necessary. The gallbladder will be removed. When my mother had hers out back in the 70s, they made a large incision. When I had mine out in 04, they did it laproscopically. Laparoscopic surgery involves making three holes and inserting a camera and then pulling the gallbladder out through the hole in the belly button area. It is painful, but recovery is usually fairly quick.

Can gallbladder disease be prevented? There does seem to be a genetic component or disposition, but there are ways to decrease your likelihood of developing it. Being overweight can be a contributing factor, so it helps to try to maintain a healthy weight. Diet is important as well. Fatty foods can be triggers, so a diet high in fiber, but low fat is recommended. Highly processed foods and refined sugars should also be avoided. Unfortunately, white rice and pasta are two of the worst foods to eat if you are at risk for gallbladder disease. High dosages of estrogen can also trigger attacks. This is why birth control and pregnancy both can be triggers as well.

Once you have your gallbladder removed, you may find that high fat foods like French fries or fried chicken, may prove to more difficult digest. I know I can only eat hamburgers, French fires and fried chicken in small amounts. A nurse at the hospital told me I wouldn't be able to eat them at all, but I found that in moderation, I am usually okay. It just important not to overdo it. Some may find that it is more difficult to digest dairy products, but I actually found it easier once my gallbladder was removed.

Chapter 22: Breast Cancer

Breast Cancer is one of the most common cancers that women get. That is why it is important to do self-exams. Although mammograms were touted as a miracle life saver in early detection, some studies show that too many mammograms may actually be contributing to cancer. While doctors still recommend getting them once you are over 40, they don't recommend getting them too often.

The causes of Breast Cancer are many. There is a strong genetic component—meaning if your mother and grandmother had it, there is a good chance you may get it as well. Now days you can get tested for the BRCA1 and BRCA2 genes. Everyone has them, but some have markers showing a defect that makes one more likely to develop cancer.

Carcinogens such as nicotine, ultraviolet rays from the sun and other environmental toxins all contribute. Smoking and drinking really do impact your health negatively. If you can't quit, cutting down will at least decrease your chances and make you feel better. Women who start menstruation early and end later have an increased chance of developing breast cancer as well. Having children and having them before age 30 can help reduce your risk. It also helps to breast feed your children when you have them.

Although oral contraceptives can decrease your cancer risk by decreasing the number of periods and length of periods, the excessive amount hormones in your system can also increase your risk. Estrogen in particular can cause problems. Some types of breast cancer are, in fact, driven by estrogen.

Being able to choose if and when you get pregnant if a great gift. It is nice to take a pill daily, get a shot or implant and forget about it. However, it seems as if the pill can cause greatly increase your likelihood of getting cancer if taken too long. It would be wise to use the pill only for short periods of time. Being on it for 10 or 20 years at a time will cause problems. And using hormone replacement after menopause should be done with great caution. Like any drug, there is a tradeoff. Women shouldn't become dependent on it when it can potentially contribute to high blood pressure, migraines and even cancer down the line.

In any case, if you get breast cancer it can be treated. If caught early, there is a high chance of becoming cancer free in the future. Options include a lumpectomy, a mastectomy and/or radiation and chemotherapy.

Chapter 23: Alternative Cancer Treatments

Cancer is a group of cells in the body that grow abnormally. There are many types of cancers, including: breast, vaginal, ovarian, cervical, pancreatic, colon, liver, stomach, lung and brain. The tumorous growths can appear in nearly any organ of the body and even in the blood. Not all cancers are alike—they can vary in size, type and cause. Historical records show that cancer has been around a long time, but it has surged in the past century—largely due to cigarette smoking and environmental toxins. There is a genetic component, but not all people with the mutated genes develop cancer and some who don't have the genetic marker will develop cancer anyway.

The signs and symptoms of cancer can vary from cancer to cancer, however, there are some things they have in common. Lumps on the skin or just under are always worth having a doctor checking out. Abnormal bleeding should never be ignored. Fatigue, loss of appetite, loss of weight and pain are common

Once a doctor had given you the diagnosis of cancer, the usual treatment consists of chemotherapy and radiation. Chemotherapy is the injection of toxins into your body to kill the cancer, but it can make you very sick. Many people who have been through chemotherapy have said they would never do it again. Radiation targets the tumor and works to slowly shrink and kill the tumor.

Sometimes, depending on where the tumor is located, surgery may be an option. Removal of the tumor is usually the only surefire way of getting rid of the cancer. And even with surgery there is no guarantee that the surgeon was able to get rid of every bit of the abnormal cells. If any of the cancer cells are left in the body the cancer may return in the same part of the body or even a different part of the body.

Currently, researchers are working on trying to understand how cancer develops and how to control it. Some theorize that the immune system can be prodded into detecting cancer and eliminating it on its own. A healthy immune system gives you better chance of keeping cancer from growing out of control. A suppressed immune system puts you at greater risk for the abnormal cells take over. That is why people with HIV/AIDS and other immune disorders need to pay closer attention to their body and any symptoms of cancer that might present them themselves.

Some doctors have found that the combination of the drugs Herceptin (trastuzumab) and Lapatinib can shrink tumors. It can be used in conjunction with chemo therapy or alone with HER2 Breast Cancer. The drug interferes with the growth of cells, but it also weakens the immune system. You have to watch out for heart and lung problems.

Letrozole us a hormone interceptor that is used in menopausal women. It can be used after tamoxifen. Tamoxifen is an antiestrogen that is used after surgery for breast cancer or chemo and radiation for breast cancer.

Nutritionists recommend the Ketogenic Diet and the use of Hyperbaric Oxygen. Some experts say that if you have cancer you should go on a high fat, medium protein and low carbohydrate diet. Dr. Gonzales also talks about using pancreatic enzyme therapy in conjunction with diet modification. However, Dr. Gerson recommends an all vegetarian diet to combat cancer risks and help in healing cancer.

The Peskin Protocol calls for the use of Omega-3 Fatty Acids that come not from fish, but from other sources. B17 is another supplement mentioned. Vitamin C and Vitamin D have also been shown to benefit those battling cancer as well.

Essiac Therapy using Essiac Tea is a controversial therapy. It uses the herbs Sheep Sorrel and Burdock Root, which are known to kill cancer cells. The other two herbs build the immune system and deal with detox and protecting the organs. However, it is most effective at the beginning stages of cancer. It isn't effective on Stage IV. Keep in mind that Essiac Tea can interact with other drugs and therapies, so use it cautiously. Diabetics and people with a blood clotting disorder may have to adjust their medication. Those who have had their gallbladder removed may not be suitable candidate for this therapy.

Iscado Therapy uses Mistletoe with Lactobacillus stimulate the immune system. Another controversial approach is to remove all mercury and silver fillings. Teeth that have had root canals are should also be removed. Baking Soda Therapy is good for digestive cancers.

Overall, you should avoid tanning beds, plastics, food additives, artificial sweeteners (aspartame) and pesticides if at all possible. Foods to eat to lower your risk: garlic, avocadoes, black seed, ginger and grapes.

Chapter 24: Ovarian Cysts

A cyst is an abnormal growth consisting of a closed cavity with liquid or semi-solid material. When an egg bursts forth from the ovary, a tiny cyst may remain. The trouble begins when the egg is trapped inside the cyst and the cyst continues to grow in size or when there are many tiny cysts covering the ovary.

Usually cysts are harmless, even if they are annoying, but sometimes they may need to be removed. If they keep increasing in size, become infected or become malignant then they might need to be removed via surgery.

Signs of an Ovarian Cyst: abdominal pain, pain during intercourse, unusual vaginal bleeding or any vaginal bleeding after menopause, unexplained weight gain or abdominal bloating, irregular periods for several months or several months no period and a negative pregnancy test, inability to become pregnant after twelve months of intercourse without birth control.

When I had intense pain on my left lower abdomen, doctors thought I had an ovarian cysts. I accepted that diagnosis and continued on with life. The pain disappeared and I didn't give it a second thought for years. Then when abdominal pain plagued me again some ten years later, another doctor suggested Polycystic Ovarian Syndrome.

Polycystic Ovarian Syndrome happens when not just one cyst appears, but many. This may happen because of an imbalance of hormones—particularly androgens. Some symptoms include menstrual irregularity, excess hair growth, acne, and obesity.

While the abdominal pain, irregularity and acne might have fit, the excess hair and obesity didn't. The doctor didn't bother to do any follow up tests, so I sought another opinion. Since then I have discovered that my pain was most likely something to do with my birth defect. This just goes to show that without extensive tests, that doctor's diagnosis is sometimes just an educated guess. If you don't think the doctor is correct, then it is your right to ask for a second opinion.

Chapter 25: Endometriosis

Another common problem that women have is endometriosis. Endometriosis happens when the lining of the uterus wanders away into other parts of the body—particularly the fallopian tubes, ovaries and abdominal cavity. Although it may sound crazy, there seems to be some truth in the ancient Greek concept of Hysteria. The Greeks once thought that women's frustration and craziness was caused by her uterus wandering throughout her body. While we now know that organs do not wander, it is possible for bits of tissue to wander.

In any case, some doctors consider it a sort of inverse or reversed flow that causes inflammation and pain. The most common symptoms of Endometriosis are heavy periods that are irregular and or heavy.

The most common treatment for Endometriosis is going on birth control. And the hormones can help lighten the flow and make periods more regular, but it isn't a permanent solutions. The combination pill with estrogen and progesterone only treats the symptoms temporarily. Some think that lower levels of progesterone may be at fault, so natural progesterone therapies might be a better long term solution.

There is also a genetic component to Endometriosis. However, Christine Northrop proposes in her book *Women's Bodies, Women's Wisdom* that Endometriosis often grows out of trauma, abuse and

caring for everybody else but yourself. The diagnosis of
Endometriosis is an opportunity to take time to care for you first and
foremost.

Chapter 26: Infertility

Getting pregnant can happen at the drop of the hat for some lucky women. For others, it can be a long and frustrating journey. I found it ironic that I spent almost ten years taking birth control and fearing getting pregnant before I was ready, but when I actually tried to conceive, it took over a year and half to do so. Not having Medicaid or medical insurance, I couldn't run to a fertility doctor and get tested either. I had no idea why it was taking so long or if I could even conceive.

This when I became an expert on fertility. The first thing to do is to check for undiagnosed Chlamydia. Not all women have symptoms. They may only be carriers, so it is important to get tested. Untreated STDs can lead to PID or Pelvic Inflammatory Disease, which can make a woman infertile. Polycystic Ovary Syndrome is another culprit in fertility problems. Uterine Fibroids can cause a lot of issues.

Fibroids are fibrous growths inside the uterus. They are noncancerous growths, but they can cause heavy periods and difficulty in getting pregnant. Usually these fibroids are noticeable in routine pelvic exams and can be treated or removed as soon as they are discovered.

If you are trying to conceive it is a good idea to take Vitamin C, Zinc, B Vitamins and Calcium to help get your body ready. Avoid drinking too much milk because that can expose you to too much galatose. And don't ignore your biological clock. Fertility drops sharply in women after 30 years old. While it is possible to get pregnant all the way up to menopause, it increasingly difficult to do so as we age. Women can get pregnant after 30 years old, but many need the help of fertility drugs and even IVF to do so.

Herbs can aid in conception, but be cautious because the same ones that may help in conception can also cause a miscarriage if used during pregnancy. Ones that are safe to use during the pregnancy period are Vitax or Chasteberry, False Unicorn's Root, Don Qui, Bupleurum and the Indian Spice Tumin. Black Cohosh can be good for regulating periods, but it can also cause miscarriages. Licorice is another herb that helps with Polycystic Ovary Syndrome, but it can cause issues during pregnancy.

Chapter 27: Fertility

Fertility is the ability to get pregnant. If you are trying to conceive, it is important to understand your cycles and be able to find out when you are ovulating. The fertile window of your cycle is only six days long total. That six day window is generally around day 10 to day 16. Some women will ovulate right after their menstrual periods or even right before their period is due, but this is the exception, not the rule.

Some women use ovulation kits to predict their fertile windows. You can also detect ovulation by paying attention to the position of your cervix. Generally the cervix is shorter and firmer between cycles. It will become longer into the vaginal canal and be softer during ovulation. If you are willing check it, it is noticeable to the touch. Then it will retract and become firmer until time for the menstrual period. When your period begins, the cervix will again become elongated and softer to the touch.

There may also be a white discharge during ovulation similar the discharge girls get before they begin menstruation. It may leave a slight stain in the underwear or be noticeable when wiping. Some women also experience ovulation bleeding as well. It isn't usually more than spotting, but it can be confusing. This ovulation spotting may make some women think they have gotten pregnant during their period when the bleeding isn't their menstrual period at all. The best way to avoid confusion is to keep track of periods and any ovulation spotting on a calendar. Be aware of what day your cycle the bleeding takes place.

Another way to know when you are ovulating is the chart your Basel body temperature. You have to check your temperature the same time every day, usually first thing in the morning, for several months to determine a pattern. When you ovulate, generally your temperature runs a little higher than normal. But first you have to establish exactly what your own normal temperature is. Illness and lack of sleep, among other things, can change your body temperature, so you need to take those things into consideration when taking your temperature each day.

Anyway, once the egg drops from the ovary and into the fallopian tube, it can last only 12 to 24 hours unless it is fertilized by the sperm. Sperm can last up to 72 hours in the uterus. Experts say it is best to have intercourse a day or two before ovulation actually takes place.

If the egg is fertilized, then about two to four days later it moves down the fallopian tube and inter the uterus, where it implants in the uterine lining. Sometimes there is a bit of spotting with the implantation and some women mistake this for an actual period. It is not a period, but it is normal.

Chapter 28: Pregnancy Tests

Home pregnancy tests have only been around since the 1970s. They've come a long way since then, but they still can't detect pregnancy from the moment of conception. Keep in mind that a pregnancy test can't detect the HCG hormone until the egg implants in the uterine wall. Even after it is implanted, the hormone levels may not be strong enough or the home test may not be sensitive enough. I've read online accounts from women who said that their pregnancy test wouldn't turn positive until the third month even though they knew that they pregnant long before that.

On the other side of that, there is the problem of so-called false positive. Although the idea of the false positive is prevalent, even among health care professionals, it seems as if it is a very rare thing indeed. If you get a positive, then most likely you are pregnant.

I know I once had a positive test and then had a very early miscarriage. I was very hurt and frustrated when the doctors and nurses at the hospital dismissed it as a mistake and said I'd merely gotten my period. I had been pregnant and I deserved a chance to grieve for what was not meant to rather than told I was mistaken—especially since my pregnancy was confirmed at the doctor's office just a few days before the miscarriage happened.

There is, however, a small possibility of misreading a test. Some of the home tests have been known to leave what they call evaporation lines, which looks like a positive, when it is in fact not a positive result at all—just a defective test. The evaporation lines occur when the pink or blue line streaks up to the top of test to show control line. The faint line may remain in the area for test result when it shouldn't. This is really the only way to get a false positive—unless of course you are man who takes the test and you have testicular cancer.

Chapter 28: Pregnancy Problems

Once the egg has implanted then the placenta forms. The corpus luteum, or the yellow tissue from the ruptured egg follicle of the ovary, continues to produce estrogen and progesterone during the pregnancy.

Hopefully your pregnancy goes smooth and is without any complications, but there are few things to look out for early on. Sometimes the egg is fertilized outside the uterine wall and this is called an Ectopic Pregnancy. The egg can start to grow either inside the fallopian tube or even on the ovary itself, but you can't carry it to term. Usually the signs of an ectopic pregnancy are: abdominal pain, abnormal bleeding, bladder or bowel problems, nausea or diarrhea, feeling light headed or faint, a missed or late period and possibly a positive pregnancy test. Generally you are either given methotrexate or surgery is done to terminate the pregnancy before it ruptures and causes internal bleeding.

Those at risk for ectopic pregnancies are those women who have had Pelvic Inflammatory Disease, Endometriosis or have been on the progesterone only pill. However, even if you have an ectopic pregnancy it is possible to conceive and carry another child to term afterward.

Another problem that can arise is the molar pregnancy. Though it is always possibility, the probability of it occurring is rare. Only about one in every 1,000 pregnancies is a molar pregnancy. This type of pregnancy occurs when a fertilized egg burrows into the lining of the uterus, but does not develop properly. The egg will grow rapidly and look like a cluster of grapes, but have no embryo inside. Essentially, the egg was defective and empty, which makes it impossible for an actual baby to grow.

How is a molar pregnancy treated? Sometimes it will spontaneously abort on its own and there is nothing else to do, but try to conceive again. Other times a D&C (dilate and curettage) is required to clean out the tissue inside the uterus.

Toxemia in another pregnancy complication. It is also known as preeclampsia. Although any pregnant woman can get it, it is more common in expectant teenagers, women over 40 or women expecting multiples. Mild Toxemia symptoms are: High blood pressure, water retention, high levels of protein in the urine, extreme weight gain, headaches, blurred vision, inability to tolerate bright lights, tiredness, nausea, vomiting, pain in the upper right abdomen, and shortness of breath. If it goes untreated, it could cause damage to the expectant mother's kidneys, brain, eyes, liver or heart. It could also cause the baby to be born smaller or prematurely. It can also lead to death for the mother and child. The only cure for preeclampsia is to deliver the baby early. If the preeclampsia is not severe or it is early in the pregnancy, efforts maybe be made to try to control the blood pressure until it is safe to deliver.

Chapter 29: Pregnancy

Trying to figure out if you are pregnant or not can be tricky since many of the symptoms are similar to PMS. Some signs are: bloating and cramps, nausea and/or vomiting, increased sense of smell, extreme fatigue, frequent urination, tender breasts, darkened areolas , Headache, heartburn, food cravings, weight gain, constipation, a missed menstrual period, spotting with implantation (light brown in color), feeling faint and even swelling of gums or tooth pain .

Nosebleeds can sometimes indicate pregnancy as well. A surge in Estrogen can cause blood vessels in the nose to swell and rupture—especially if it is winter and you are in dry air in a lot. This increase in blood volume increases means you need to increase your intake of folic acid and iron pregnancy.

Women gain weight during pregnancy as well, but only a small fraction of that is the baby. Up to 25% of weight gain is due increased fluids throughout the body. If there is an excess of swelling and fluid though, the doctor may recommend cutting down on salt or sodium. Sometimes the fluid buildup may result in issues like carpel tunnel syndrome, but usually it is not a problem. You might try dandelion root to help with fluid retention since it is a diuretic.

It is also important to pay attention to the list of medications that are approved to take during pregnancy. Many things will be off limits during this time, but it is okay to take something mild like Tylenol for aches and pains. They say to avoid Advil because it can cause or contribute to bleeding. Benadryl is probably one of the safest drugs to take during pregnancy. Sudafed and Actifed can only be used after 12 weeks and only if your doctor approves it. If you have high blood pressure, decongestants can make it worse. Metamucil and Colace are safe to take for constipation. Tums, Maalox and Mylanta are safe for indigestion. Yeast infections can be a problem during pregnancy. Monistat and Gyne-Lotrimin can be used.

Some women are lucky to not feel sick at all, but others feel sick from morning to night through most of their pregnancy. Aside from nibbling on crackers to settle your stomach, you can also drink herbal tea. Chamomile, Red Raspberry, Peppermint and Ginger are all herbs that help with nausea. Other herbs you can take during pregnancy are: Nettles, Bilberry, Burdock Root, Yellow Dock Root, Don Qui Root, Echinacea, Wild Yam, False Unicorn's Root, Dandelion and Alfalfa.

Be careful though, there are a number of herbs that are dangerous to take during pregnancy. Herbs to avoid during pregnancy are: Aloe Vera, Angelic, Rue, Barberry, Buckhorn, Rhubarb Root, Black Cohosh, Comfrey, Ephedra, Ma Huang, Buchu and Juniper, Horseradish, Goldenseal, Male Fern, Mistletoe, Pennyroyal, Yarrow and Shepherd's Purse.

Chapter 30: Labor and Delivery

Once you've made it through your pregnancy then it will come time to go into labor. Lamaze class is recommended for preparation for the big event. Early signs of labor include: the baby dropping lower, the cervix dilating, cramping and increased back pain. Your vaginal discharge changes color and consistency. Joints may feel looser, you may have diarrhea, weight gain may stop or you might even lose weight, there may be an extra-tired feeling or having an urge to nest.

Labor usually begins with the onset of consistent contractions, but you may lose your mucus plug or have your water break before contractions begin. Sometimes the doctors will have to break your water for you if it doesn't break before, but that is usually a last resort.

Preterm labor occurs when regular contractions begin to open your cervix before 37 weeks of pregnancy. A full-term pregnancy should last about 40 weeks. Signs of preterm labor are very similar to regular labor, except that the contractions may start off as mild cramping. If preterm labor can't be stopped, your baby will be born early. The earlier that the premature birth happens, the greater the health risks for the baby.

There is a great deal of controversy over the use of drugs during labor. While many feel it is better for the baby for the mother not to use any sort of drugs during labor, others feel that it really doesn't do any harm. I can tell you that I felt very strongly about having a natural childbirth, but once my labor stalled several hours in I changed my mind. I got the epidural and was able to rest before my daughter was born. I don't regret it. In fact, when in to deliver my son, I asked for the epidural right away. The truth is, it is a personal choice and you shouldn't feel pressured either way. Do what you feel is best for you and your baby.

An Episiotomy is the when the doctor cuts the peritoneal tissue between the vaginal and anal opening. This practice become common years ago and still done in some hospitals. It was believed that a surgical cut was safer than a tear. However, the cut goes through muscle tissue and is often more severe than natural superficial tears.

There is also a lot of heated discussion about natural childbirth versus having a C-section. Natural childbirth is certainly best, if possible, but there are many times that a C-section is medically necessary, like for breech births. I've had both a natural childbirth and a C-section. The natural birth took longer labor wise, but the recovery time was much shorter. The C-section was medically necessary for me since my son was breech. My labor was much shorter with the C-section, which was nice, but the recovery time was much longer.

Chapter 31: Breastfeeding

It used to be that women were discouraged from breastfeeding. Around WWI and WWII women were given bottles and told that it was better to use those. You could know exactly how much your baby was eating and could make sure that they had the proper nutrition from scientifically made formula. Then in the late sixties and early seventies, things began to swing the other way. Women began choosing to breastfeed despite the fact that many doctors and nurses advised them not to. Now women are encouraged to breastfeed if at all possible.

So why Breastfeed? Well, women who breastfeed have less bleeding after childbirth ad lose weight sooner. Breastfeeding women also have less risk of breast, ovarian and uterine cancer. They also have stronger bones.

Colostrum is the thick yellowish milk that comes in first. It is a miracle food for babies because it is the perfect balance of nutrients of what babies need. It prepares the baby's system for healthy digestion, and helps babies pass their first bowel movement. Colostrum is full of antibodies that fight germs and it builds immunity.

Breastfed babies have fewer infections, have less risk of allergies and asthma, have less constipation and diarrhea, have less risk of

SIDS, have less risk of childhood obesity, and have less risk for diabetes.

Breasts were made for feeding babies and it is best for them if you can breastfeed, but there are many reasons a mother may chose not to breastfeed. Problems with the baby latching on properly, engorgement, lack of milk, lack of time and mastitis or a breast infection are all reasons why a woman may not be able to breastfeed her baby.

I wanted to feed my daughter, but I was unable to at first. She was a preemie and the doctors and nurses wanted me to give her a high calorie formula and measure how much she was eating. I had to pump and freeze my milk, which was not fun. After a few weeks of this frustrating practice, I was able to begin nurse her, and I continued nursing her for a long time after that.

How long you breastfeed is up to you as a mother, but infants need either formula or breast milk for the first year. They will be on a diet of milk exclusively for about three months and then you can slowly introduce baby food. The American Pediatric Association recommends breastfeeding for at least 6 to 12 months. The Le Leche League recommends at least 12 to 24 months, but they are quick to say that you should breastfeed long you are comfortable with breastfeeding. Though not common, it is not unheard of for a mother to breast feed until their child is 3 or 4 years old. Some mothers believe in child led weaning, while other feel that as soon as they feel ready that they are going to wean the child themselves. Either is fine because it is a personal choice.

Studies show that the longer you breastfeed your baby, the smarter and more well-adjusted they will be. DHA, or Docosahexaenoic Acid, is an omega-3 fatty acid that is a primary structural component of the human brain, cerebral cortex, skin, and retina is important for the baby's development. Most formulas have taken to adding this important ingredient into their mix, but it occurs naturally in your breast milk.

As an adult you can take DHA supplements as well. In fact, it is suggested by some that you take DHA throughout your pregnancy and while you are breastfeeding.

Chapter 32: Breastfeeding Safety

You have to be very careful about what you eat and what herbs and drugs you take during pregnancy. You also have to watch what you eat and take while you are breastfeeding.

Common Over the Counter Drugs you can take while breastfeeding include: Aleve for short term use, Tylenol, and Advil that is 400 milligram or less. Aspirin should be used with caution, as it can cause Reyes Syndrome in your baby. Antacids are generally safe, but plain baking soda should be avoided. Antidiarrheal Medication is okay, but you have to be cautious with Pepto Bismol as it an aspirin based product. Aspartame—also known as Equal or NutraSweet—is also aspirin based and should be avoided while breastfeeding. Sweet and Low is Saccrin, but should probably not be used either.

Non-drowsy cold and cough medicine is okay. However, anything with a an antihistamine should be used with caution. If it makes you sleepy, it may also make your baby sleepy. It can also decrease your milk supply.

Laxatives are to be used with caution. Glycerin Suppositories, Colace and Metamucil are safe, but Exlax and similar products could cause pain and colic in your nursing baby.

Dramamine and similar products for motion sickness are okay to take. However, the safety of Dramaminell, Marezine, Bonine have not been determined.

Caffeine in small doses is safe for mother and baby, but more than 150 milligrams a day could cause your baby to be irritable and have an upset stomach. Coffee has 115 milligrams of caffeine, while tea only has 60 milligrams of caffeine. Iced tea, however, can have up to 70 milligrams of caffeine. Coca-Cola has about 45 milligrams of caffeine, while Pepsi has about 38 milligrams. Mountain Dew has a whopping 54 milligrams of caffeine in it. So, nursing mothers should limit themselves to one cup of coffee or two sodas a day. Vivarin has too much caffeine in it and should be avoided.

Breastfeeding is a natural way to lose weight. Talking weight loss products while nursing can be dangerous to both you and your baby. These products often have high levels of caffeine in addition to other potentially harmful ingredients. Please wait until you are finished breastfeeding to take any weight loss products.

If you have to have an outpatient procedure done it is safe for a nursing mother to be injected with anesthetics such as midazolam, propofol and thiopental. These drugs leave the system pretty quickly and so by the time a mother is ready to nurse again, it should be out of her system. Local anesthetics such as Novocain are also safe to be used on mothers who are breastfeeding.

Penicillin and other mild antibiotics are safe to take while breastfeeding. In fact, doctors will give infants and toddlers penicillin directly to deal with ear infections and the like. However, clindamycin, Isoniazid, metronidazole should not be used while nursing. Tetracyclines are generally not given to children, pregnant or nursing women because they can stain an infant's teeth.

Anticoagulants such as heparin, enoxaparin and dalteparin are acceptable to mothers who are breastfeeding, but only in small amounts. Anticonvulsants do pass into breast milk and should be taken with caution during breastfeeding. Phenobarbital has been given directly to infants for years without adverse effects. Antifungals are, for the most part, safe to take. Clotirmazole has actually been used on infants directly when they suffer from thrush. Ketoconazole should not be applied to a nursing mother's nipples though. It could be toxic to the baby. The antivirals Acyclovir, Famciclovir and Calaciclovir are safe to take. Amantadine, which is often used to treat the flu, is not safe to use during breastfeeding.

Ergotamine, which is often used to treat migraines, should not be used while nursing. Narcotics can be used while breastfeeding, but they can cause drowsiness in infants. Asthma medications and inhalers are safe to use, but only is small amounts. Diuretics are also safe to use, but only in small doses. They can decrease milk production.

Heart and blood pressure medication is not often used during pregnancy and lactation, but most of the drugs are thought to be relatively safe. Amiodarone one of the few heart medicines known to cause low thyroid levels and has delayed growth in breastfeeding infants and should not be taken.

Antidiabetic drugs are fairly safe, but a nursing mother may need to lower her dosage right after birth. The combination birth control pills, which contain both estrogen and progesterone should not be taken while breastfeeding. Estrogen is known to suppress milk production. Progesterone only pills are often prescribed to nursing mothers, but only after the first six weeks. Corticosteroids can be taken while breastfeeding, but only in small dosages.

Alcohol should not be consumed in large quantities while breastfeeding, as it passes through the breast milk and cause your baby to become drunk. An occasional drink probably won't cause any harm, but you should wait two hours after drinking to nurse. Marijuana use during breastfeeding can have adverse effect as well. Heavy use can lead to infants with delayed muscular development and coordination. Cocaine and Crack are very toxic to infants and should never be used during pregnancy or breastfeeding either one.

Smoking cigarettes while nursing can increase your baby's risk for colic, RSVP and SIDS. It is suggested that smokers try to quit, cut down or use nicotine patches and gum. Not only does nicotine pass into your milk, but the second hand smoke can cause issues as well.

Mood tranquillizers and antidepressants can have some effects in nursing infants, but not much is known about their long term effects. Most notably, doxepin and similar drugs can make your baby drowsy. Postpartum depression can adversely affect your baby's growth and development, so sometimes doctors will decide the risk of prescribing the drugs is acceptable compared to the severity of your postpartum depression. Fluoxetine or Prozac is one the few antidepressants to cause colic and digestive upsets in nursing babies. Citalopram can appear in high amounts in breast milk, so it is not ideal to take. Sertraline or Zoloft us safer to take. Lithium is dangerous to take while breastfeeding because high amounts of it can pass through the breast milk and accumulate in your baby's bloodstream.

Chapter 33: WIC

WIC stands for Mothers, Infants and Children. **WIC** was formally created by an amendment to section 17 of the Child Nutrition Act of 1966 on September 26, 1972. It was created to help mothers with low income to get the nutrition that they needed to have a healthy pregnancy and raise healthy children.

If you get food stamps or are on Medicaid, you will be eligible for WIC. However, sometimes if you on the just above the poverty line and can't get food stamps, you may still be able to get WIC. That was the case with my first pregnancy.

Once you get accepted, WIC will issue an EBT card, which is like a debit card, or paper vouchers. These coupons will be for milk, cheese and juice. They also help with breastfeeding support or the purchase of formula if you can't breastfeed. If want to breastfeed, but have to return to work they often provide you with an electric breast pump.

WIC will have you attend classes on nutrition and do check-ups on you and you your baby. They will check on weight and blood pressure as well as test your baby's blood for lead levels during your visits.

WIC is a wonderful resource and has lots of newsletters, pamphlets and information for you to draw on. They are very supportive and can connect you other agencies if they can't help you with a particular issue or situation.

Chapter 34: Co-Sleeping

Co-sleeping is the term used when a mother and father will bring the baby into the family bed. Although this practice was common at one time, it felt out of favor. Mothers were told to put their baby in a crib in another room so they could have privacy and get some sleep.

Since families have been choosing co-sleeping in the face of modern convention, there has been much controversy over it. The biggest concern, other than lack of privacy, is that the parents will roll over and suffocate the baby in the middle of the night. Studies show that that most parents will innately avoid rolling over on their child. The only time that this is truly a concern is if the parents have been drinking or doing drugs. Alcohol and drugs suppress this natural inclination or intuition to keep the baby safe. If you don't drink or do drugs, then this shouldn't be a problem. However, the American Pediatric Association likes to err on the side of caution and recommends not sleeping with your baby in the same bed as you—just in case.

On the positive side of co-sleeping, there is chance to bond with your baby and also the convenience of letting the baby breastfeed on demand. Exhausted mothers find it easier to bring the baby to bed rather than breastfeed in a sitting up in a chair and putting it back in the bassinette or crib and returning to bed. They may leave the baby in their bed on purpose, but many have simply fallen asleep along with their baby during the feeding. Rather co-sleeping is choice or something that just happened naturally, it up to you.

An alternative to co-sleeping would be to simply keep the baby in the same room as you and your partner. A bassinette or crib in your bedroom will be more convenient than having to go to another room for the first few months and it eliminates the concern over accidental smothering.

Chapter 35: Coping With Colic

What is Colic? Colic is the term used to describe uncontrollable crying in an otherwise healthy baby. If your baby is younger than 5 months old and cries for more than three hours in a row on three or more days a week for at least three weeks (phew!), he or she is considered colicky. If you feed them, change them and hold them and they are still crying, it is probably colic. Dr. Harvey Karp lays out some very good advice on how to deal with colic in his book *The Happiest Baby on the Block.*

The first thing Karp recommends is swaddling. Your baby was used to being confined in the womb, and for the first couple months outside the womb, he or she misses that security. You can wrap the baby tightly in a blanket when they are fussy in order to calm them. Their arms and legs will be bound, but their heads should remain free. Although you can lay them in their crib or bassinette like this, it works best if you hold them and carry them during this time. After they are calm and happy, you should unwrap them or loosen the blanket so they can move around better.

Sucking is also soothing to your baby. Whether it is sucking on a nipple to feed or sucking on a pacifier, the act of sucking came calm your baby. If you baby refuses to feed or use a pacifier and is still fussy, you can try propping them on their side rather than letting them lay on their back or their stomach. You can also position them sideways on your shoulder or lap if you want. This may help with gas and/or indigestion or simply be a nice change that makes them more comfortable.

Saying shush in a quiet, calming voice may aid in calming your baby, but keep in mind that your tone is important. If you don't want to keep saying shush, you can trying calming white noises— like say a fan. Some mothers play CDs or download MP3s of white noise or lullabies and play them when their baby is fussy.

Swinging is another tool. You can gently swing them from side to side in your arms while you are holding them or you can put them in a baby swing. Your baby felt you move around all day for nine months, so it misses that constant movement. If you can replicate that gentle, but constant movement, you can sooth your baby.

Sometimes just changing your formula or changing your diet when you are breastfeeding can eliminate the gas and pain. This may help with frequent crying. If that doesn't help there are Gas Drops can help crying or colic associated with indigestion. I found that the natural Gripe Water works better than the simethicone gas drops. There are many types of Gas Drops for babies out there. Finding out what one works for you and your baby is usually a matter of trial and error.

Chapter 36: Infant to Toddler Feeding

Continue iron fortified formula or breastfeeding until the baby's first birthday. They baby shouldn't drink whole cow's milk until after one year. And make sure they drink the milk from a cup, not a bottle. A baby can start to drink from a cup at 5 or 6 months old. And limit Juice to 4 ounces a day and out of cup. Never a Bottle. Juice dampens your child's appetite. Deserts should be offered sparingly since they have very little nutrition.

4-7 Months: Feed a Single Ingredient. Food First: Infant Cereals, Vegetables and Fruits. 7-9 Months: Infants are leaning to put things in their mouths. They may ready for finger foods, which will dissolve in their mouths. 10-18 Months: They can eat soft meats: Meatballs and Sauce, Ground Beef or Ground Turkey, Water Packed Tuna, Fish without Bones, Fish Sticks, Chicken Nuggets, and Tender Pork Chops with No Bones, Tender Roast Beef and Ham with no Bone. They can also eat Grains: Baked French Fries, Tator Tots, Cooked Cereals, and Toasted Bagels Cut up into Small Pieces, Biscuits, Pretzel Sticks, and Cookies. Dairy Products: Mild Cubed Cheese, Cottage Cheese, Yogurt, Ice Cream, Custard and Pudding. Vegetables: Soft cooked broccoli or cauliflower, tomatoes, peeled cucumber, mushrooms, green peppers, baked beans and Brussels Spouts. Fruits: Orange sections, strawberries, grapes cut in half, soft melons, fruit cocktails, crushed pineapple.

Make sure you don't give your toddler a food they can't chew. That is why you should cut their food into little bits. Teach your toddler to chew and swallow before speaking. Talking with a mouthful isn't just rude, but a choking hazard. A child who is choking may not make any sound at all, so listen for silence. Don't let your children run while they are eating, as this is also a choking hazard.

Let your child decide when he or she is full. Stop feeding them when they show you that they've had enough. Signs to watch for are: turning their head away, spitting food out, playing with the food or is distracted by other people or things.

Introduce new foods one at a time to avoid allergic reactions. Then feed the baby the same food for 3-5 days in a row to make sure.

Food Dangers include: fish with bones, whole hot dogs, whole grapes, cherry tomatoes, chewy meats, hard candy, popcorn, nuts, olives, raisins, potato chips, peanut butter, gum, fruits with seeds, raw carrots, raw celery, whole peas and whole green beans, seeds, marshmallows and large chunks of any foods.

Chapter 37: Food Storage

Although many of us have gotten into the bad habit of thawing food on the kitchen counter, it is better to thaw them in the refrigerator instead. Slower thawing will prevent the loss of moisture and the lower temperature thawing will keep bacteria from growing. Food that has been thawed generally cannot be refrozen and should be tossed.

Your freezer should always be at 0 degrees Fahrenheit or 32 degree Celsius for optimum results. At 0 degrees or below, your freezer will prevent bacteria from multiplying. Once the food is thawed out, bacteria is free to grow again though. This is why it is vital to make sure any meat you cook is cooked thoroughly so you don't get sick. Your refrigerator should be set to 40 degrees or below. When cooking, the food should be heated to 140 degrees or higher to make sure the bacteria is killed. Meat thermometers can help you determine if your dish is cooked if you have any concerns.

Bacteria is the cause of 67 percent of the food poisoning in the US. There are three types of bacteria responsible for food poisoning. Staphylococcus, Clostridium Perfrigins and Salmonella. Although these bacteria are commonly found in our food they don't cause problems until they have been given a chance to multiply and take over the food we wish to eat. Moisture and heat are conducive to bacteria growth, which is why we keep many things in the fridge or the freezer to keep.

How long does food last in the freezer and fridge? Good question! Meats like bacon, ground beef, ground pork and similar meats last between 1 month and 3 months. Lunch meat can last 3 to 12 months in the freezer. Fish can last up to 6 months in the freezer. However, breaded fish, king crab, lobster tails, oysters and other seafood is only good for about 2 to 3 months.

Fruits that are frozen can last up to a year. Citrus fruit and fruit juice concentrates only last for about 6 months though. Vegetables that you freeze or that you purchase already frozen are good for about 8 to 10 months in your freezer.

Cakes, casseroles and cookies can be frozen and stay good up 3 months in your freezer. Unbaked pies can stay good up to 8 months in the freezer. Nuts that are salted or unsalted can last between 6 to 12 months. Generally salted nuts last longer, as salt is a preservative.

Dairy Products like butter and margarine can be frozen and held for 6 to 12 months. Buttermilk, sour cream and yogurt should never be frozen. Cheese, however, is good to be frozen for about 3 months. It should be thawed in the fridge and never at room temperature though. Do not freeze eggs in their shells. Out of the shell the whites and yolks can last up to a 12 months. Ice cream and sherbet are okay in your freezer for up to two months. Milk can be frozen and stay good for up to a month in the freezer as well.

Always thaw milk in the refrigerator and never at room temperature though.

Vegetables need to be kept at 37 degrees or lower in the fridge. Lettuce only keep for 3 to 5 days before turning brown and going bad. Ripe tomatoes only last a couple of days as well. Uncooked meat lasts 1 to 3 days in the fridge before needing to be tossed. Cured and smoked meats can last 2 to 7 days in the fridge. Canned goods put in the fridge can last 2 days to 1 week maximum.

Canned foods have a long shelf life, but they do not last indefinitely. Even if they do not make you sick, old canned foods may not taste very good. Keep an eye out for bulging cans because that usually means the food inside has spoiled. Dented cans can mean that the can isn't sealed properly and the food could be bad or go bad quicker than normal. Rusty cans could mean the food or juice is leaking.

Bread keeps fresh at room temperature and usually good for a week or two. Brown breads and other high moisture breads should be stored in the fridge. If it is hot and humid out, consider putting your bread in the fridge to prevent mold growth. However, refrigerated bread has a tendency to go stale quicker.

Flour should be stored in an airtight container. It should be kept at room temperature unless it is very hot and humid, in which case, you can put small amounts in the fridge or freezer to keep. Brown Sugar often dries out into blocks so hard that you need a hammer to break them. It is best to warm it slowly on a cookie sheet in the oven (250 to 300 degrees max) and then put it in an airtight container once cool and soft.

Dry onions and potatoes prefer to be in cool, dark places. Onions and potatoes may sprout, so only buy enough for the week. If you buy too much and it spouts after a while, then toss it. Do not refrigerate sweet potatoes. Unripe tomatoes and peaches may be left out until ripe and then placed within the refrigerator. Apples should be stored some place below 60 degrees. Bananas are generally left out of the fridge because the cold causes them to turn brown quicker.

White Flour lasts 6 to 8 months. Baking Powder and Baking Soda can last 18 months to 2 years in the cupboard. Sugars generally last about 4 months. Bouillon cubes can last up to 2 years if kept dry and covered. Cereals—unopened—have a shelf life of about 6 to 12 months. Chocolate for cooking keeps about 12 months as long as it is kept cool. Chocolate Syrup is good 6 months to 2 years unopened. Coca Mixes are only good up to 8 months. So that mix from two years ago should be tossed! Coffee lasts about a 2 years unopened. Instant coffee will only last about 1 year unopened. Opened coffee will only last 2 weeks to 2 months. So drink up.

Honey doesn't really go bad exactly, but it won't taste near as good after 12 months. Jellies and Jams should be used up during 12 months as well. Mayonnaise will last 2-3 months unopened. After is opened, it should be refrigerated. Salad Dressings will last 10-12 months unopened. Once you open them, they are only good for about 3 months. Ketchup and Chili Sauce will be fine unopened for a year, but only about 1 month after opening. Mustard will last up to 2 years unopened and only about 6 to 8 months opened. Spices and herbs will last anywhere from 6 months to 2 years depending on if they are whole or ground and if they are in air tight containers.

Pastas that are held in airtight containers and remain uncooked can last for up to 2 years. Rice can last from 6 months to 2 years, but it is important to keep the package tightly closed. Mixed and Packaged foods such as instant potatoes, soup mixes and rice mixes will stay good 6 to 12 months.

Cake mixes are good for about 9 to 12 months. However, if you purchased a cake already made it will only last about 1 to 2 days before it will need to be tossed. Cookies can last two to three weeks once made. Packaged cookies bought at the store will last about two months if the package is airtight or unopened. Crackers will last 3 months in airtight boxes and packages. Pancake Mix will only last about 6 to 9 months. Pie Crust mixes will last about 8 months.

Chapter 38: Yoga

Yoga has been around for centuries in India, but really only been taught in the US for a little over 60 years. Though it was taught in the 1960s, it become mainstream until the 1980s. Today Yoga is taught nearly everywhere—from private studios to Recreation Centers to YMCAs.

Hatha Yoga is the most commonly practiced form of Yoga. Hatha means willful or forceful and Yoga means to yoke, connect or unite. Yoga poses are called Asanas. Hatha Yoga utilizes a series of poses or stretches to help strengthen the body and quiet the mind. Iyengar Yoga is usually a lot more active and demanding than Hatha Yoga.

Pranayama Yoga focuses on breathing exercises. This Yoga focuses on Mediation and helps with relaxation, but it can also help asthma and other breathing issues. There are other types of Yoga that don't rely on poses or asanas like Karma Yoga. Karmic Yoga is the practice of selfless service to humanity whereby a spiritual seeker attempts to give their actions selflessly without hoping for rewards or recognition. Bhakti Yoga is a spiritual path or spiritual practice within Hinduism focused on the cultivation of love and devotion toward God or the Goddess.

The great thing about Yoga is that you can enjoy it regardless of what you believe or don't believe. Christian, Hindu, Buddhist or Wiccan—it doesn't matter what you are. Yoga is for all.

In any case, physical practice of Yoga has many benefits, including: increased flexibility, increased muscle strength and tone, improved respiration, energy and vitality, maintaining a balanced metabolism, weight reduction, cardio and circulatory health, improved athletic performance and protection from injury.

I've been doing Yoga since about 1999 and I love it. I've found it to be very important to my life. I return from class less stressed and feeling a bit more centered. Usually I only manage to go once a week, but I couldn't definitely see it being beneficial to go five days a week or more. It has also kept me flexible and in good shape.

When I injured my back and had to go for physical therapy, the physical therapist was amazed at my range of motion. My lower back, which was what I had injured, was the only thing that really needed worked on. Everything else was in good shape. Most of the people she saw in physical therapy often had severely limited range of motion and weren't very flexible at all.

The great thing about Yoga is that is one physical activity that you can do during pregnancy as well. However, for the first trimester you really need to take at easy and focus on meditation. Once you are into the second and third trimesters, you have a lot more freedom in your movements. Some modifications must be made, but so long as feel up to, I highly recommend yoga during pregnancy. It is a good idea to find a yoga instructor who will work with you modifying poses or find a class specifically tailored to expectant moms.

Chapter 39: Goddesses For Women's Health

Geraldine Gardner is considered the founding father of modern Wicca which draws heavily upon pagan deities and traditions. Traditionally the Wiccan Goddesses are known in the form of the triple goddess: the mother, the maiden and the crone. One of the most common symbols of the Wicca is the triple moon, combining the images of the waxing, full and waning moon. Celtic, Egyptian, Norse, Greek and Roman Goddesses are often referred to, but other deities may be included.

Arianrhod (Celtic) - Goddess of fertility, rebirth and the weaving of cosmic time and fate. The last aspect of her nature is contained within her name which means "silver wheel" or "round wheel," suggesting her importance in the cycles of life.

Asherah (Canonite) Ancient goddess mentioned in the Old Testament. She is a fertility goddess and known as the maiden, mother and crone.

Bast (Egyptian) - The famous cat Goddess, she protected pregnant woman and children. Bast was a very sensual Goddess who enjoyed music, dance and perfume. Her name comes from the bas jars used to store perfumes and ointments.

Freya (Nordic) - Goddess of love, beauty, fertility, war, wealth, divination and magic. Her name comes from the ancient Norse word for lady or mistress.

Frigg (Nordic) - Goddess of marriage, childbirth, motherhood, wisdom, household management and weaving and spinning. Her name means "beloved" in ancient Norse and is derived from fri "to love."

Hathor (Egyptian) - This heavenly cow's areas of influence included music, dancing, joy and fertility. Her name translates as "house of Horus".

Hera (Greek) - Queen of the Olympians and Goddess of marriage and birth. The meaning of her Goddess name has been lost. One historian claims her name could be connected to the Greek word for seasons "hora," suggesting she is ripe for marriage.

Hestia (Greek) Goddess of the home and hearth. She is a virgin goddess in charge of ordering of domesticity, the family, the home, and the state. Her name means fireside.

Inanna (Sumerian) - Goddess of love, war, and fertility. Inanna was the personification of the morning and evening star. Her beautiful name means "lady of the sky." This Goddess is closely linked to Ishtar and Nin-anna.

Juno (Roman) - Goddess of marriage, pregnancy and childbirth. She protected the finances of the citizens of Rome. Her name is mystery, it speaks of a contradictory role for this Goddess, before her alignment to the matronly, Greek Goddess, Hera. This is because her name is derived from the root yeu meaning "vital force" indicating a more youthful, maiden Goddess.

Ostara (Germanic) - The spring Goddess whose name is linked to the East and the dawn. The early Christians took her fertility symbols of eggs and hares and incorporated them into the Easter celebrations.

Rhea (Greek) - The ancient Titan Earth Goddess, responsible for the fertility of the soil and women. The name is most likely a form of the word era meaning "earth", although it has also been linked to 'rheos' the Greek term for "stream."

Works Consulted

Anatomy of the Spirit, Carolyn Myss, 1997.

Food Storage Website https://whatscookingamerica.net/ Information/FreezerChart.htm

Misconceptions, Naomi Wolfe, 2001.

Hypoglycemia: The Disease Your Doctor Won't Treat,
　　Saunders and Ross, *1980.*

Planned Parenthood Website
https://www.plannedparenthood.org/

Our Bodies, Ourselves, Boston Women's Health Collective,
　　1976.

The Grain Brain, Brian Pearlmutter, 2013.

The A to Z Guide to Healing Herb Remedies, Elias and
　　Masline, 1995.

The Feminine Mystic, Betty Friedan, 1964.

The Happiest Baby on The Block, Dr. Harvey Karp, 2002.

The Le Leche League Website: http://www.lalecheleague.org/

The Low Blood Sugar Handbook: Edward and Patricia
　　Krimmel, 1992.

The Mayo Clinic Website, http://www.mayoclinic.org/

The Yeast Connection, William G Crook, 1984.

Three In A Bed: The Benefits of Sleeping With Your Baby, Debora Jackson, 2003.

Woman: An Intimate Geography, Natalie Angier, 1999.

Women's Bodies, Women's Wisdom, Christine Northrup, 1998

www.ingramcontent.com/pod-product-compliance
Lightning Source LLC
Chambersburg PA
CBHW062037280526
45788CB00003B/1029